Vegetarian Diet Cookbook 2021

The Best Beginner's Guide to Cook and Enjoy Affordable & Tasty Vegetarian Recipes for a Best Life

Natalie Clark

Table of Content

Breakfasts

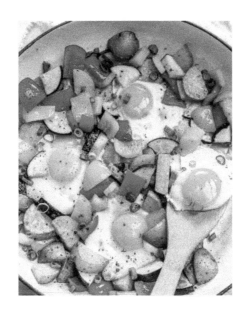

Healthy Breakfast Bowl

Preparation time: 10 m

Cooking time: 10 m

Ingredients:

1 vegan yogurt

1/2 avocado (peeled and diced)

1 handful blueberries

1 tablespoon cacao nibs

1 handful of strawberries

1 tablespoon mulberries

1 tablespoon goji berries

1 tablespoon desiccated coconut

Directions:

Put the avocado in a nice bowl.

Top up with vegan yogurt.

Sprinkle the remaining ingredients and enjoy it.

Nutrition: carbohydrates: 55 g calories: 471 Fat: 25g sodium: 183 g protein: 11 g sugar: 32 g

Oatmeal Raisin Breakfast Cookie

Preparation time: 5 minutes

Cooking time: 15 minutes

Servings: 2 cookies

Ingredients

½ Cup rolled oats

1 tablespoon whole-grain flour

½ Teaspoon baking powder

1 to 2 tablespoons brown sugar

½ Teaspoon pumpkin pie spice or ground cinnamon (optional)

¼ Cup unsweetened applesauce, plus more as needed

2 tablespoons raisins, dried cranberries, or vegan chocolate chips

Directions

In a medium bowl, stir together the oats, flour, baking powder, sugar, and pumpkin pie spice (if using). Stir in the applesauce until thoroughly combined. Add another 1 to 2 tablespoons of applesauce if the mixture looks too dry (this will depend on the type of oats used).

Shape the mixture into 2 cookies. Put them on a microwave-safe plate and heat on high power for 90 seconds.

Alternatively, bake on a small tray in a 350°f oven or toaster oven for 15 minutes. Let cool slightly before eating.

Nutrition (2 cookies): calories: 175; protein: 74g; total fat: 2g; saturated fat:0g; carbohydrates: 39g; fiber: 4g

Root Vegetable Hash With Avocado Crème

Preparation time: 25 m

Cooking time: 10 m

Ingredients:

1/2 c onion, diced

1 T vegan butter

2 cloves garlic, minced

1 c sweet potatoes, diced

1 c turnips, diced

1 c broccoli florets, diced

2 vegan sausages, diced

1 c collard greens, chopped

1/2 tsp sea salt

1 tsp cumin

1/2 tsp black pepper

1/4 – 1/2c vegetable stock

1/4 c fresh cilantro, chopped

1 medium avocado

1 T balsamic vinegar

1/4 c cashews

Directions:

Melt and hest the butter in a skillet. Add onion and garlic and sauté until they are translucent about 5 minutes.

Add sweet potatoes and turnips stir to match. Cook for 5-8 minutes.

Add the broccoli and vegetables. Continue cooking until it turns light green and start to soften for 5 to 8 minutes.

Add the roasted field, salt, pepper, cumin, coriander, and vinegar. Reduce the heat and get it cooked until the meat is hot and the flavors melt.

Mix the avocado, cashews, and vegetable broth in a blender until smooth.

Plate and serve with a spoonful of avocado cream on top. Garnish with more cilantro.

Nutrition: 19 g fat 30 g of carbohydrates 17 g protein 7 g sugar 691 mg sodium

Country Breakfast Cereal

Preparation Time: 5 minutes

Cooking time: 40 minutes

Servings: 6

 Ingredients:

1 cup brown rice, uncooked

½ cup raisins, seedless

1 tsp cinnamon, ground

¼ Tbsp peanut butter

2 ¼ cups water

Honey, to taste

Nuts, toasted

Directions:

Combine rice, butter, raisins, and cinnamon in a saucepan.

Add 2 ¼ cups water. Bring to boil.

Simmer covered for 40 minutes until rice is tender.

Fluff with fork. Add honey and nuts to taste.

Nutrition: Calories 160 Carbohydrates 34 g Fats 1.5 g Protein 3 g

Blueberry Oat Muffins

Preparation time: 10 minutes

Cooking time: 20 minutes

Servings: 12 muffins

Ingredients

2 tablespoons coconut oil or vegan margarine, melted, plus more for preparing the muffin tin

1 cup quick-cooking oats or instant oats

1 cup boiling water

½ Cup nondairy milk

¼ Cup ground flaxseed

1 teaspoon vanilla extract

1 teaspoon apple cider vinegar

1½ cups whole-grain flour

½ Cup brown sugar

2 teaspoons baking soda

Pinch salt

1 cup blueberries

Directions

Preheat the oven to 400°f.

Coat a muffin tin with coconut oil, line with paper muffin cups, or use a nonstick tin.

In a large bowl, combine the oats and boiling water. Stir so the oats soften. Add the coconut oil, milk, flaxseed, vanilla, and vinegar and stir to combine. Add the flour, sugar, baking soda, and salt. Stir until just combined. Gently fold in the blueberries. Scoop the muffin mixture into the prepared tin, about ⅓ cup for each muffin.

Bake for 20 to 25 minutes, until slightly browned on top and springy to the touch. Let cool for about 10 minutes. Run a dinner knife around the inside of each cup to loosen, then tilt the muffins on their sides in the muffin wells so air gets underneath. These keep in an airtight container in the refrigerator for up to 1 week or in the freezer indefinitely.

Nutrition (1 muffin): calories: 174; protein: 5g; total fat: 3g; saturated fat:2g; carbohydrates: 33g; fiber: 4g

Orange French Toast

Preparation time: 15 minutes

Cooking time: 10 minutes

Servings: 4

Ingredients

3 very ripe bananas

1 cup unsweetened nondairy milk

Zest and juice of 1 orange

1 teaspoon ground cinnamon

¼ Teaspoon grated nutmeg

4 slices french bread

1 tablespoon coconut oil

Directions

In a blender, combine the bananas, almond milk, orange juice and zest, cinnamon, and nutmeg and blend until smooth. Pour the mixture into a 9-by-13-inch baking dish. Soak the bread in the mixture for 5 minutes on each side.

While the bread soaks, heat a griddle or sauté pan over medium-high heat. Melt the coconut oil in the pan and swirl to coat. Cook the bread slices until golden brown on both sides, about 5 minutes each. Serve immediately.

Oatmeal Fruit Shake

Preparation Time: 10 minutes

Cooking time: 0 minutes

Servings: 2

Ingredients:

1 cup oatmeal, already prepared, cooled

1 apple, cored, roughly chopped

1 banana, halved

1 cup baby spinach

2 cups coconut water

2 cups ice, cubed

½ tsp ground cinnamon

1 tsp pure vanilla extract

Directions:

Add all ingredients to a blender.

Blend from low to high for several minutes until smooth.

Nutrition: Calories 270 Carbohydrates 58 g Fats 1.5 g Protein 5 g

Chocolate Strawberry Almond Protein Smoothie

Preparation time: 10 m

Cooking time: 10 m

Ingredients:

1 cup of organic strawberries

1 1/2 cup homemade almond milk

1 scoop chocolate protein powder

1 tablespoon organic coconut oil

1/4 cup organic raw almonds

1 tablespoon organic hemp seeds

1 tablespoon organic maca powder

For Garnish:

organic cacao nibs

organic hemp seeds

Directions:

Put all the ingredients inside a blender and beat until they are well combined.

Optional: Garnish with organic hemp seeds or organic cocoa beans.

Enjoy it!

Nutrition: carbohydrates: 39 g calories: 720 Fat: 45 g sodium: 732g protein: 44 g sugar: 12g

Amaranth Banana Breakfast Porridge

Preparation Time: 10 minutes

Cooking time: 25 minutes

Servings: 8

Ingredients:

2 cup amaranth

2 cinnamon sticks

4 bananas, diced

2 Tbsp chopped pecans

4 cups water

Directions:

Combine the amaranth, water, and cinnamon sticks, and banana in a pot. Cover and let simmer around 25 minutes. Remove from heat and discard the cinnamon. Places into bowls, and top with pecans.

Nutrition: Calories 330 Carbohydrates 62 g Fats 6 g Protein 10 g

Berry Beetsicle Smoothie

Preparation time: 3 minutes

Cooking time: 0minutes

Servings: 1

Ingredients

½ Cup peeled and diced beets

½ Cup frozen raspberries

1 frozen banana

1 tablespoon maple syrup

1 cup unsweetened soy or almond milk

Directions

Combine all the Ingredients in a blender and blend until smooth.

Entrées

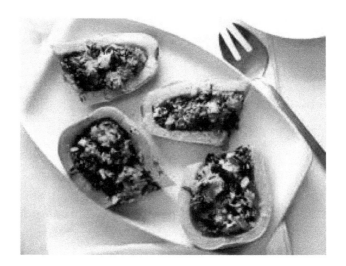

Homemade Trail Mix

Preparation time: 20 minutes Cooking time: 20 minutes

Servings: 2

Ingredients:

½ cup uncooked old-fashioned oatmeal

½ cup chopped dates

2 cups whole grain cereal

¼ cup raisins

¼ cup almonds

¼ cup walnuts

Directions: Mix all the ingredients in a large bowl.

Place in an airtight container until ready to use.

Nut Butter Maple Dip

Preparation time: 1 hour

Cooking time: 1 hour

Servings:

Ingredients:

½ tablespoon ground flaxseed

1 teaspoon ground cinnamon

½ tablespoon maple syrup

2 tablespoons cashew milk

¾ cups crunchy, unsweetened peanut butter

Directions:

In a bowl, combine the flaxseed, cinnamon, maple syrup, cashew milk and peanut butter.

Use a fork to mix everything in. I stir it like I'm scrambling eggs. The mixture should be creamy. If it's too runny, add a little more peanut butter; if it's too thick, add a little more cashew milk.

Refrigerate for about an hour, covered and serve.

Soups, Salads, and Sides

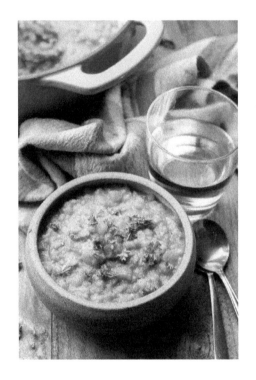

The Amazing Chickpea Spinach Salad

Preparation time: 10 mins

Cooking time: 10 mins

Ingredient: 1 can chickpeas (drained and rinsed)

   1 handful spinach

   3.5 oz feta cheese (or similar cheese)

   1 small handful raisins

   ½ tbsp lemon juice (white or malt vinegar is also good)

   3 tsp honey

   4 tbsp olive oil

   0.5 - 1 tsp cumin

   1 pinch salt

   ½ tsp chili flakes (or dried cayenne pepper will do the trick nicely).

Directions: Chop the cheese and add with the spinach and chickpeas to a large bowl

Mix the honey, oil, lemon juice and raisins in a small bowl. Add the cumin, salt and pepper to the dressing bowl and mix well. Drizzle devilishly delicious dressing over the salad.

Tamari Toasted Almonds

Preparation time: 2 minutes

Cooking time: 8 minutes

Servings: ½ cup

Ingredients:

½ cup raw almonds, or sunflower seeds

2 tablespoons tamari, or soy sauce

1 teaspoon toasted sesame oil

Directions:

Preparing the ingredients.

Heat a dry skillet to medium-high heat, then add the almonds, stirring very frequently to keep them from burning. Once the almonds are toasted, 7 to 8 minutes for almonds, or 3 to 4 minutes for sunflower seeds, pour the tamari and sesame oil into the hot skillet and stir to coat.

You can turn off the heat, and as the almonds cool the tamari mixture will stick to and dry on the nuts.

Nutrition: calories: 89; total fat: 8g; carbs: 3g; fiber: 2g; protein: 4g

Chickpea, Red Kidney Bean And Feta Salad

Preparation time: 5 mins

Cooking time: 5 mins

Ingredient:

   1 can chickpeas

   1 can red kidney beans

   1 piece small of ginger grated or shredded

   1 medium onion diced

   2- 3 cloves garlic

   1   tbsp olive oil

   A pinch of red chili flakes

   3-4 spring onions green part only, chopped, scallions

   1 cup chopped parsley OR coriander I used cilantro

   Juice of one lemon

   150 g feta cheese – almost half cup size

   Salt and Black pepper.

Directions:

Heat 1 tablespoon of olive oil and cook the onion till lightly golden. Do not overdo it and the onions should still be crunchy. Add garlic, ginger and chili and cook till the garlic is fragrant. Set aside to cool so it doesn't melt the feta when you mix it in. Drain the chickpeas and red kidney beans, rinse and place in the salad bowl. Add crumbled feta, spring onion, parsley (or coriander) and lemon juice, season with salt and pepper. Add the cooled onion and garlic mixture and remaining oil and mix well.

Marinated Mushroom Wraps

Preparation time: 15 minutes

Cooking time: 0 minutes

Servings: 2 wraps

 Ingredients:

3 tablespoons soy sauce

3 tablespoons fresh lemon juice

1½ tablespoons toasted sesame oil

2 portobello mushroom caps, cut into ¼-inch strips

1 ripe hass avocado, pitted and peeled

2 cups fresh baby spinach leaves

1 medium red bell pepper, cut into ¼-inch strips

1 ripe tomato, chopped

Salt and freshly ground black pepper

Directions:

In a medium bowl, combine the soy sauce, 2 tablespoons of the lemon juice, and the oil. Add the portobello strips, toss to combine, and marinate for 1 hour or overnight. Drain the mushrooms and set aside.

Mash the avocado with the remaining 1 tablespoon of lemon juice.

To assemble wraps, place 1 tortilla on a work surface and spread with some of the mashed avocado. Top with a layer of baby spinach leaves. In the lower third of each tortilla, arrange strips of the soaked mushrooms and some of the bell pepper strips. Sprinkle with the tomato and salt and black pepper to taste. Roll up tightly and cut in half diagonally. Repeat with the remaining ingredients and serve.

Lunch Recipes

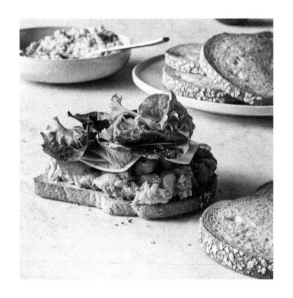

Simple Curried Vegetable Rice

Preparation Time: 30 Minutes

Cooking Time: 10 Minutes

Servings: 4

Ingredients:

Carrots (2, Chopped)

Spinach (1 C., Chopped)

Ginger (2 t.)

Broccoli (1, Chopped)

Salt (to Taste)

Cooked Brown Rice (1 C.)

Garlic (2, Minced)

Pepper (to Taste)

Curry Powder (1 t.)

Directions:

Before you begin cooking, you will want to take some prep time to chop up all of your vegetables beforehand. When they are cut into smaller pieces, this means they will cook faster! Once your ingredients are prepared, take out a pan and begin to heat it over a medium heat. Once warm, add in some olive oil and then sprinkle in the garlic and the ginger.

Next, you will want to add in the broccoli and carrots. At this point, season with salt and pepper and cook for two minutes. Once the vegetables are cooked to your liking, add in the cooked brown rice along with the curry powder and toss the ingredients until everything is well coated.

Finally, add in the spinach and cook for another minute or until it becomes wilted. Season with some more salt and pepper, and then your meal will be ready just like that!

Nutrition: Calories: 280 Proteins: 10g Carbs: 50g Fats: 5g

Black Bean And Bulgur Chili

Preparation Time: 10 minutes

Cooking Time: 20 minutes

Serving: 4

Ingredients:

3/4 cup (177 grams) bulgur wheat, ground

30 ounces (850 grams) cooked black beans

1 medium red bell pepper, cored, diced

1 red onion, peeled, chopped

1 medium green bell pepper, cored, diced

1 chipotle pepper in adobo sauce, deseeded, diced

1 teaspoon minced garlic

1 teaspoon smoked paprika

1/8 teaspoon sea salt

1 teaspoon dried oregano

1 teaspoon ground cumin

3 cups (710 ml) vegetable broth

1 tablespoon olive oil

1 lime, juiced

1 ¼ cups (295 grams) enchilada sauce

For Topping:

1/2 cup (118 grams) chopped cilantro

Directions:

Take a large pot, place it over medium-low heat, add oil and when hot, add onion and garlic, season with salt, and cook for 3 minutes until softened.

Add bell peppers, continue cooking for 5 minutes until tender, add remaining ingredients and stir until mixed.

Bring the mixture to a boil, switch heat to a low level and simmer for 10 minutes.

Taste to adjust seasoning, then remove the pot from heat, cover it with lid and let it stand for 10 minutes.

Distribute chili among bowls, top with cilantro and serve.

Nutrition: 387 Cal; 6.5 g Fat; 1.2 g Saturated Fat; 67.5 g Carbs; 18.6 g Fiber; 19.8 g Protein; 6 g Sugar;

Buffalo Cauliflower Wings

Preparation Time: 30 Minutes

Cooking Time: 15 Minutes

Servings: 4

Ingredients:

Chickpea Flour (.75 C)

Almond Milk (1 C.)

Buffalo Sauce (1 C.)

Cauliflower (1 Head)

Curry Powder (1 t.)

Onion Powder (1 t.)

Garlic Powder (1 t.)

Nutritional Yeast (2 T.)

Directions:

You will want to begin this recipe by prepping the oven to 450. As this warms up, go ahead and prep a baking sheet with parchment paper and then set it to the side.

Next, you are going to take a bowl and combine the nutritional yeast and spices with the flour.

With your flour made up, carefully dip the cauliflower into the soymilk and directly into the flour. Once the cauliflower piece is well coated, place it onto your baking sheet and continue until you have covered every cauliflower floret.

When you are ready, pop the baking dish into the oven for about twenty minutes. After this time, the cauliflower should be crispy.

Once the cauliflower is cooked through, place it into a bowl, and toss with the hot sauce. When all of the pieces are well coated, place them back into the oven for another ten minutes, and then they will be ready.

Nutrition: Calories: 160 Proteins: 11g Carbs: 20g Fats: 3g

Arugula and Artichokes Bowls

Preparation time: 5 minutes

Cooking time: 0 minutes

Servings: 4

Ingredients:

2 cups baby arugula

¼ cup walnuts, chopped

1 cup canned artichoke hearts, drained and quartered

1 tablespoon balsamic vinegar

2 tablespoons cilantro, chopped

2 tablespoons olive oil

Salt and black pepper to the taste

1 tablespoon lemon juice

Directions:

In a bowl, combine the artichokes with the arugula, walnuts and the other ingredients, toss, divide into smaller bowls and serve for lunch.

Nutrition: calories 200, fat 2, fiber 1, carbs 5, protein 7

Minty arugula soup

Preparation time: 5 minutes

Cooking time: 10 minutes

Servings: 4

Ingredients:

3 scallions, chopped

1 tablespoon olive oil

½ Cup coconut milk

2 cups baby arugula

2 tablespoons mint, chopped

6 cups vegetable stock

2 tablespoons chives, chopped

Salt and black pepper to the taste

Directions:

Heat up a pot with the oil over medium high heat, add the scallions and sauté for 2 minutes.

Add the rest of the ingredients, toss, bring to a simmer and cook over medium heat for 8 minutes more.

Divide the soup into bowls and serve.

Nutrition: calories 200, fat 4, fiber 2, carbs 6, protein 10

Thai Tofu And Quinoa Bowls

Preparation Time: 15 minutes

Cooking Time: 20 minutes

Serving: 4

Ingredients:

3/4 cup (177 grams) quinoa, cooked

1 cup (236 grams) frozen edamame, thawed

12 ounces (175 grams) tofu, extra-firm, pressed

2 medium carrots, grated

1 green onion, sliced

1/2 teaspoon minced garlic

2 teaspoons grated ginger

1/2 cup chopped cilantro

1/2 teaspoon red chili flakes

1 tablespoon soy sauce

2 teaspoons agave syrup

2 tablespoons lime juice

2 tablespoons peanut butter

1 tablespoon water

4 teaspoons sesame seeds, toasted

Directions:

Switch on the oven, set it to 400° F and let it preheat.

Prepare the tofu: cut tofu into ¾-inch cubes.

Take a large baking sheet, line it with foil, spread tofu pieces on it, and bake for 20 minutes until golden brown, stirring halfway.

Prepare the drizzle: take a small bowl, place garlic, ginger, chili flakes, soy sauce, agave syrup, butter, lime, and water in it and then whisk until combined.

After tofu gets cooked, let it cool for 10 minutes and transfer into a large bowl.

Add carrot, green onions, cilantro, cabbage, and edamame, drizzle with the prepared dressing and sprinkle with sesame seeds.

Mix quinoa with salad and serve.

Nutrition: 330 Cal; 13 g Fat; 3 g Saturated Fat; 36 g Carbs; 7 g Fiber; 19 g Protein; 10 g Sugar;

Spicy Southwestern Hummus Wraps

Preparation Time: 15 Minutes

Cooking Time: 0 Minutes

Servings: 1

Ingredients:

Whole-wheat Wrap (1)

Lettuce (1 C., Shredded)

Tomato (1 T., Diced)

Hummus (4 T.)

Avocado (2 T., Diced)

Corn (2 T.)

Black Beans (2 T.)

Directions:

For a quick lunch, simply lay out your wrap and spread the hummus over the surface. Once the hummus is in place, layer the rest of the ingredients and then roll the wrap up before eating.

Nutrition: Calories: 400 Proteins: 15g Carbs: 50g Fats: 15g

Dinner Recipes

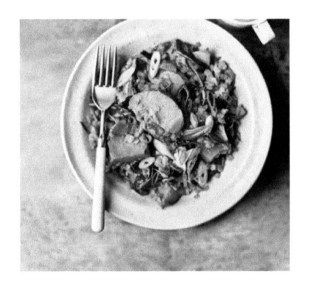

Pistachio Watermelon Steak

Preparation Time: 5 min.

Cooking Time: 10 min.

Servings: 4

Ingredients:

Microgreens

Pistachios chopped

Malden sea salt

1 tbsp. olive oil, extra virgin

1 watermelon

Salt to taste

Directions:

Begin by cutting the ends of the watermelon.

Carefully peel the skin from the watermelon along the white outer edge.

Slice the watermelon into 4 slices, approximately 2 inches thick.

Trim the slices, so they are rectangular in shape approximately 2 x4 inches.

Heat a skillet to medium heat add 1 tablespoon of olive oil.

Add watermelon steaks and cook until the edges begin to caramelize. Plate and top with pistachios and microgreens. Sprinkle with Malden salt.

Serve warm and enjoy!

Nutrition: Calories: 67 | Carbohydrates: 3.8 g | Proteins: 1.6 g Fats: 5.9 g

Spicy Veggie Steaks With Veggies

Preparation Time: 30 min.

Cooking Time: 45 mins.

Servings: 4

Ingredients:

1 ¾ c. vital wheat gluten

½ c. vegetable stock

¼ t. liquid smoke

1 tbsp. Dijon mustard

1 t. paprika

½ c. tomato paste

2 tbsp. soy sauce

½ t. oregano

¼ t. of the following:

coriander powder

cumin

1 t. of the following:

onion powder

garlic powder

¼ c. nutritional yeast

¾ c. canned chickpeas

Marinade:

½ t. red pepper flakes

2 cloves garlic, minced

2 tbsp. soy sauce

1 tbsp. lemon juice, freshly squeezed

¼ c. maple syrup

For skewers:

15 skewers, soaked in water for 30 minutes if wooden

¾ t. salt

8 oz. zucchini or yellow summer squash

¼ t. ground black pepper

1 tbsp. olive oil

1 red onion, medium

Directions:

In a food processor, add chickpeas, vegetable stock, liquid smoke, Dijon mustard, pepper, paprika, tomato paste, soy sauce, oregano, coriander, cumin, onion powder, garlic, and natural yeast. Process until the ingredients are well-mixed. Add the vital wheat gluten to a big mixing bowl, and pour the contents from the food processor into the center. Mix with a spoon until a soft dough is formed.

Knead the dough for approximately 2 minutes; do not over knead.

Once the dough is firm and stretchy, flatten it to create 4 equal-sized steaks.

Individually wrap the steaks in tin foil; be sure not to wrap the steaks too tightly, as they will expand when steaming.

Steam for 20 minutes. To steam, you can use any steamer you like or a basket over boiling water.

While steaming, prepare the marinade. In a bowl, whisk the red pepper, garlic, soy sauce, lemon juice, and syrup. Reserve half of the sauce for brushing during grilling.

Prepare the skewers. Cut the onion and zucchini or yellow squash into 1/2-inch chunks.

In a glass bowl, add the red onion, zucchini, and yellow squash then coat with olive oil, pepper, and salt to taste. Place the vegetables on the skewers.

After the steaks have steamed for 20 minutes, unwrap and place on a cookie sheet. Pour the marinade over the steaks, fully covering them.

Bring your skewers, steaks, and glaze to the grill. Place the skewers on the grill over direct heat. Brush skewers with glaze. Grill for approximately 3 minutes then flip.

Place the steaks directly on the grill, glaze side down, and brush the top with additional glaze. Cook to your desired doneness.

Serve warm and enjoy!

Nutrition: Calories: 458 | Carbohydrates: 65.5 g | Proteins: 39.1 g | Fats: 7.6 g

Curry Mushroom Pie

Preparation Time: 65 minutes

Cooking Time: 1 hour

Servings: 4

Ingredients:

For the piecrust:

1 tbsp flax seed powder + 3 tbsp water

¾ cup plain flour

4 tbsp. chia seeds

4 tbsp almond flour

1 tbsp nutritional yeast

1 tsp baking powder

1 pinch salt

3 tbsp olive oil

4 tbsp water

For the filling:

1 cup chopped baby Bella mushrooms

1 cup vegan mayonnaise

3 tbsp + 9 tbsp water

½ red bell pepper, finely chopped

1 tsp curry powder

½ tsp paprika powder

½ tsp garlic powder

¼ tsp black pepper

½ cup coconut cream

1¼ cups shredded vegan Parmesan cheese

Directions:

In two separate bowls, mix the different portions of flaxseed powder with the respective quantity of water. Allow soaking for 5 minutes.

For the piecrust:

Preheat the oven to 350 F.

When the flax egg is ready, pour the smaller quantity into a food processor and pour in all the ingredients for the piecrust. Blend until soft, smooth dough forms.

Line an 8-inch springform pan with parchment paper and grease with cooking spray.

Spread the dough in the bottom of the pan and bake for 15 minutes.

For the filling:

In a bowl, add the remaining flax egg and all the filling's ingredients. Combine well and pour the mixture on the piecrust. Bake further for 40 minutes or until the pie is golden brown.

Remove from the oven and allow cooling for 1 minute.

Slice and serve the pie warm.

Bbq Ribs

Preparation Time: 30 min.

Cooking Time: 45 min.

Servings: 2

Ingredients:

2 drops liquid smoke

2 tbsp. of the following:

soy sauce

tahini

1 c. of the following:

water

wheat gluten

1 tbsp. of the following:

garlic powder

onion powder

lemon pepper

2 t. chipotle powder

For the Sauce:

2 chipotle peppers in adobo, minced

1 tbsp. of the following:

vegan Worcestershire sauce

lemon juice

horseradish

onion powder

garlic powder

ground pepper

1 t. dry mustard

2 tbsp. sweetener of your choice

5 tbsp. brown sugar

½ c. apple cider vinegar

2 c. ketchup

1 c. water

1 freshly squeezed orange juice

Directions:

Set the oven to 350 heat setting, and prepare the grill charcoal as recommended for this, but gas will work as well.

Combine soy sauce, tahini, water, and liquid smoke in a bowl. Then set this mixture to the side in a mixing bowl.

Next, use a big glass bowl to mix chipotle powder, onion powder, lemon pepper, garlic powder; combine well then whisk in the ingredients from the little bowl.

Add the wheat gluten and mix until it comes to a gooey consistency.

Grease a standard-size loaf pan and transfer the mixture to the loaf pan. Smooth it out so that the rib mixture fits flat in the pan.

Bake for 30 minutes.

While the mixture is baking, make the BBQ sauce. To make the sauce, combine all the sauce ingredients in a pot. Allow the mixture to simmer its way to the boiling point to combine the flavors, and as soon as it boils, decrease the heat to the minimum setting. Let it be for 10 more minutes.

Cautiously take the rib out of the oven and slide onto a plate.
Coat the top rib mixture with the BBQ Sauce and place on the
grill.

Coat the other side of the rib mixture with BBQ Sauce and grill
for 6 minutes

Flip and grill the other side for an additional 6 minutes.

Serve warm and enjoy!

Nutrition: Calories: 649 | Carbohydrates: 114 g | Proteins: 34.8
g | Fats: 11.1g

Smoothies, Snacks and Desserts

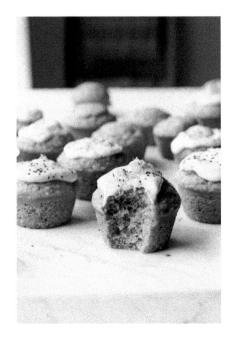

Pumpkin Chia Smoothie

Preparation Time: 5 Minutes

Cooking Time: 0 minutes

Serves: 1

Calories: 726

Protein: 5.5 Grams

Fat: 69.8 Grams

Carbs: 15 Grams

Ingredients:

3 Tablespoons Pumpkin Puree

1 Tablespoon MCT Oil

¾ Cup Coconut Milk, Full Fat

½ Avocado, Fresh

1 Teaspoon Vanilla, Pure

½ Teaspoon Pumpkin Pie Spice

Directions:

Combine all ingredients together until blended.

High Protein Avocado Guacamole

Preparation time: 15 minutes

Cooking time: 0 minutes

Servings: 4

Ingredients

1/2 cup of onion, finely chopped

1 chili pepper (peeled and finely chopped)

1 cup tomato, finely chopped

Cilantro leaves, fresh

2 avocados

2 Tbsp linseed oil

1/2 cup ground walnuts

1/2 lemon (or lime)

Salt

Directions:

Chop the onion, chili pepper, cilantro, and tomato; place in a large bowl.

Slice avocado, open vertically, and remove the pit.Using the spoon take out the avocado flesh.Mash the avocados with a fork and add into the bowl with onion mixture.Add all remaining ingredients and stir well until ingredients combine well.Taste and adjust salt and lemon/lime juice.

Keep refrigerated into covered glass bowl up to 5 days.

Vegan Eggplant Patties

Preparation time: 30 minutes

Cooking time: 15 minutes

Servings: 6

Ingredients

2 big eggplants

1 onion finely diced

1 Tbsp smashed garlic cloves

1 bunch raw parsley, chopped

1/2 cup almond meal

4 Tbsp Kalamata olives, pitted and sliced

1 Tbsp baking soda

Salt and ground pepper to taste

Olive oil or avocado oil, for frying

Directions

Peel off eggplants, rinse, and cut in half.

Sauté eggplant cubes in a non-stick skillet - occasionally stirring - about 10 minutes.

Transfer to a large bowl and mash with an immersion blender.

Add eggplant puree into a bowl and add in all remaining ingredients (except oil).

Knead a mixture using your hands until the dough is smooth, sticky, and easy to shape.

Shape mixture into 6 patties.

Heat the olive oil in a frying skillet on medium-high heat.

Fry patties for about 3 to 4 minutes per side.

Remove patties on a platter lined with kitchen paper towel to drain.

Serve warm.

Green Soy Beans Hummus

Preparation time: 15 minutes

Cooking time: 0 minutes

Servings: 6

Ingredients

1 1/2 cups frozen green soybeans

4 cups of water

coarse salt to taste

1/4 cup sesame paste

1/2 tsp grated lemon peel

3 Tbsp fresh lemon juice

2 cloves of garlic crushed

1/2 tsp ground cumin

1/4 tsp ground coriander

4 Tbsp extra virgin olive oil

1 Tbsp fresh parsley leaves chopped

Serving options: sliced cucumber, celery, olives

Directions:

1. In a saucepan, bring to boil 4 cups of water with 2 to 3 pinch of coarse salt.

2. Add in frozen soybeans, and cook for 5 minutes or until tender.

3. Rinse and drain soybeans into a colander.

4. Add soybeans and all remaining ingredients into a food processor.

5. Pulse until smooth and creamy.

6. Taste and adjust salt to taste.

7. Serve with sliced cucumber, celery, olives, bread...etc.

Kale & Avocado Smoothie

Preparation Time: 10 Minutes

Cooking time: 0 minute

Servings: 1

Ingredients:

1 ripe banana

1 cup kale

1 cup almond milk

¼ avocado

1 tbsp. chia seeds

2 tsp. honey

1 cup ice cubes

Direction:

Blend all the ingredients until smooth.

Nutrition: Calories 343 Total Fat 14 g Saturated Fat 2 g
Cholesterol 0 mg Sodium 199 mg Total Carbohydrate 55 g
Dietary Fiber 12 g Protein 6 g Total Sugars 29 g Potassium
1051 mg

Mango And Banana Shake

Preparation time: 10 mins

Cooking time: 0 mins

Servings: 2

Ingredients:

1 Banana, Sliced And Frozen

1 Cup Frozen Mango Chunks

1 Cup Almond Milk

1 Tbsp. Maple Syrup

1 Tsp Lime Juice

2-4 Raspberries For Topping

Mango Slice For Topping

Directions

In blender, pulse banana, mango with milk, maple syrup, lime juice until smooth but still thick

Add more liquid if needed.

Pour shake into 2 bowls.

Top with berries and mango slice.

Enjoy!

Nutrition: Protein: 5% 8 kcal Fat: 11% 18 kcal Carbohydrates: 85% 140 kcal

Coconut & Strawberry Smoothie

Preparation Time: 10 Minutes

Cooking Time: 0 minutes

Serves: 1

Calories: 278

Protein: 14 Grams

Fat: 2 Grams

Carbs: 57 Grams

Ingredients:

1 Cup Strawberries, Frozen & Thawed Slightly

1 Ripe Banana, Sliced & Frozen

½ Cup Coconut Milk, Light

½ Cup Vegan Yogurt

1 Tablespoon Chia Seeds

1 Teaspoon Lime juice, Fresh

4 Ice Cubes

Directions:

Blend everything together until smooth, and serve immediately.

Granola bars with Maple Syrup

Preparation time: 15 minutes

Cooking time: 0 minutes

Servings: 12

Ingredients

3/4 cup dates chopped

2 Tbsp chia seeds soaked

3/4 cup rolled oats

4 Tbsp Chopped nuts such Macadamia, almond, Brazilian...etc,

2 Tbsp shredded coconut

2 Tbsp pumpkin seeds

2 Tbsp sesame seeds

2 Tbsp hemp seeds

1/2 cup maple syrup (or to taste)

1/4 cup peanut butter

Directions:

Add all ingredients (except maple syrup and peanut butter) into a food processor and pulse just until roughly combined.

Add maple syrup and peanut butter and process until all ingredients are combined well.

Place baking paper onto a medium baking dish and spread the mixture.

Cover with a plastic wrap and press down to make it flat.

Chill granola in the fridge for one hour.

Cut it into 12 bars and serve.

Keep stored in an airtight container for up to 1 week.

Also, you can wrap them individually in parchment paper, and keep in the freezer in a large Ziploc bag.

Homemade Energy Nut Bars

Preparation time: 15 minutes

Cooking time: 0 minutes

Servings: 4

Ingredients

1/2 cup peanuts

1 cup almonds

1/2 cup hazelnut, chopped

1 cup shredded coconut

1 cup almond butter

2 tsp sesame seeds toasted

1/2 cup coconut oil, freshly melted

2 Tbsp organic honey

1/4 tsp cinnamon

Directions

Add all nuts into a food processor and pulse for 1-2 minutes.Add in shredded coconut, almond butter, sesame seeds, melted coconut oil, cinnamon, and honey; process only for one minute.Cover a square plate/tray with parchment paper and apply the nut mixture.Spread mixture vigorously with a spatula.Place in the freezer for 4 hours or overnight.Remove from the freezer and cut into rectangular bars.

Ready! Enjoy!

Avocado Toast With Flaxseeds

Preparation time: 5 mins. Cooking time: 0 mins

Servings: 3

Ingredients:

3 slice of whole grain bread

1 large avocado, ripe

¼ cup chopped parsley

1 tbsp. flax seeds

1 tbsp. sesame seeds

1 tbsp. lime juice

Directions:

First, toast your piece of bread.

Remove the avocado seed.

Slice half avocado and mash half avocado with fork in bowl.

Spread mashed avocado on 2 toasted bread.

Place avocado slice on 1 toast.

Top with flax seeds and sesame seeds.

Drizzle lime juice and chopped parsley on top.Serve and enjoy!

Nutrition: Protein: 12% 31 kcal Fat: 49% 124 kcal

Carbohydrates: 39% 98 kcal

Cantaloupe Smoothie Bowl

Preparation Time: 5 Minutes

Cooking Time: 0 minutes

Serves: 2

Calories: 135

Protein: 3 Grams

Fat: 1 Gram

Carbs: 32 Grams

Ingredients:

¾ Cup carrot Juice

4 Cps Cantaloupe, Frozen & Cubed

Mellon Balls or Berries to Serve

Pinch Sea Salt

Directions:

Blend everything together until smooth.

Vegan Breakfast Sandwich

Preparation Time: 10minutes

Cooking Time: 10 minutes

Servings: 3

Ingredients

1 tsp. coconut oil

6 slices of bread

1 14 oz container

1-2 tsp. vegan

extra firm tofu

mayo

1 tsp. turmeric

1 cup of greens

1/2 tsp. garlic

1-2 medium

powder

tomatoes

1/2 tsp. Kala

6 pickle slices

Namak (black

Fresh cracked

salt)

pepper

3 melty vegan
cheese slices

Directions:

Season one facet of the tofu with salt, garlic powder, break up pepper, and turmeric. I just 15 sprinkled it out of the flavor bins. You will season the second side within the field when it is a perfect possibility to flip them.

In a medium skillet, warmth oil over medium warmth and notice the tofu cuts organized aspect down on the dish. While the bottom facet is cooking, season the pinnacle side. Let the tofu cook dinner for three to 5 minutes, till marginally darker and clean. Presently turn the cuts over and fry the alternative aspect for 3-5 minutes. Presently's a respectable time to pop the bread in the toaster, on every occasion liked.

To liquefy the cheddar, on a preparing sheet, place 2 cuts of tofu one next to the opposite, with a reduce of cheddar over every set. Put it within the broiler on prepare dinner for 1-three minutes, until the cheddar is dissolved. You can likewise utilize a toaster broiler.

Spread mayo on the two aspects of the bread.

Spot the two cuts of tofu with cheddar on one aspect. Include the vegetables and tomatoes.

Presently include several pickle cuts and near the sandwich collectively. Cut nook to corner

Chickpea And Mushroom Burger

Preparation Time: 20minutes

Cooking Time: 16 minutes

Serving: 4

Ingredients

240g chickpeas

Half tsp. sea salt

2 level tsp. gram

Half medium-

flour

sized apple

1 small red

1 tsp. dried

onion

parsley

2 large cloves

1 tsp. fresh

garlic

rosemary

75g tasty

1 medium-sized

mushrooms

tomato

1 tsp. tahini

Directions

Pulverize garlic, diced onion and slash the mushrooms into little pieces; saute together in a search for a gold couple of moments.

Generally, pound chickpeas in an enormous blending bowl in with a potato masher or fork. The pound doesn't need to be absolutely smooth, in spite of the fact that you do need to give it a decent squeezing through with the goal that a great deal of it is very soft. It's fine to leave a couple of provincial looking pieces.

Mesh the half apple.

Include the gram flour, tahini, salt, and apple and combine all utilizing the rear of a metal spoon

Finely cleave the rosemary and slash the tomato into little pieces.

Include the sauteed things alongside every single residual ingredient into a bowl, pushing down and blending completely with a metal spoon.

Partition into 4 and solidly shape and form into patties.

Spot onto a barbecue plate and warmth under a medium flame broil for roughly 8 minutes on each side.

Flavour Boosters and Souce Recipes

Mexican Cocoa Rub

Want to spice up your dry meats with savory Mexican flavors? Try out my classy rub this weekend. Cocoa and espresso powder are a special addition to this Mexican style rub creating soothing spiced aroma.

Preparation Time: 5 min.

Cooking Time: 5 min.

Servings: 9 tsp.

Ingredients:

Water – 1 tbs.

Cocoa, unsweetened – 1 tsp.

Instant espresso powder – 2 tsp.

Smoked paprika – 2 tsp.

Olive oil – 1 tsp.

Ground cumin – 1 tsp.

Salt – ¼ tsp.

Directions:

One by one, mix in all the ingredients in your mixing bowl to make the cocoa rub. Gently mix all the ingredients using spatula or spoon to form an aromatic rub mixture.

Now, take your choice of meat cut and place it on a firm surface. Brush or rub the freshly made rub on it; pat gently for the rub to stick to the surface. Turn the meat cut and repeat to spice up its other side. Repeat with other meat cuts.

Let your meat cuts adequately season for more rich flavors for a few hours in your refrigerator. Take them out, as they are ready to be cooked or grilled!

Juniper Sage Meat Rub

This unique meat rub has been crafted with quality by including numerous healthy herbs such as juniper berries, lay leaf, red pepper, etc. It delivers piney accent to the rub, which ultimately enhances the flavor of your favorite meat cuts.

Preparation Time: 5 min.

Cooking Time: 5 min.

Servings: 8 tsp.

Ingredients:

Bay leaf - 1

Black peppercorns - 1 tsp.

Juniper berries - 2 tsp.

Extra-virgin olive oil - 2 tbs.

Crushed red pepper - ½ tsp.

Kosher salt - ½ tsp.

Minced garlic – 1 clove

Minced sage leaves – 6

Directions:

Mix in the bay leaf, red pepper, salt, peppercorns, and berries in your spice blender, grinder or processor to make the juniper rub. Start processing or grinding the mixed spiced on "pulse" mode to ground.

Empty the mixed spice mixture in a bowl; mix in the sage leaves, oil, and garlic. Mix again well.

Now, take your choice of meat cut and place it on a firm surface. Brush or rub the freshly made rub on it; pat gently for the rub to stick to the surface. Turn the meat cut and repeat to spice up its other side. Repeat with other meat cuts.

The freshly rubbed meat is ready to be grilled or cooked!

Coconut Sugar Peanut Sauce

Preparation time: 5 minutes

Cooking time: 5 minute

Servings: 1 ½ cups

Ingredients

4 tablespoons coconut sugar

6 tablespoons powdered peanut butter

1 tablespoon chili sauce

2 tablespoons liquid aminos

¼ cup of water

1 teaspoon lime juice

½ teaspoon ginger powder

Directions:

In a bowl, combine all the ingredients until properly combined. Serve as a topping for the salad or other dishes. Store in a fridge.

Meal Plans

Meal Plan 1

Day	Breakfast	Lunch	Dinner	Snacks
1	Chocolate PB Smoothie	Cauliflower Latke	Noodles Alfredo with Herby Tofu	Beans with Sesame Hummus
2	Orange french toast	Roasted Brussels Sprouts	Lemon Couscous with Tempeh Kabobs	Candied Honey-Coconut Peanuts
3	Oatmeal Raisin Breakfast Cookie	Brussels Sprouts & Cranberries Salad	Portobello Burger with Veggie Fries	Choco Walnuts Fat Bombs
4	Berry Beetsicle Smoothie	Potato Latke	Thai Seitan Vegetable Curry	Crispy Honey Pecans (Slow Cooker)
5	Blueberry Oat Muffins	Broccoli Rabe	Tofu Cabbage Stir-Fry	Crunchy Fried Pickles

6	Quinoa Applesauce Muffins	Whipped Potatoes	Curried Tofu with Buttery Cabbage	Granola bars with Maple Syrup
7	Pumpkin pancakes	Quinoa Avocado Salad	Smoked Tempeh with Broccoli Fritters	Green Soy Beans Hummus
8	Green breakfast smoothie	Roasted Sweet Potatoes	Cheesy Potato Casserole	High Protein Avocado Guacamole
9	Blueberry Lemonade Smoothie	Cauliflower Salad	Curry Mushroom Pie	Homemade Energy Nut Bars
10	Berry Protein Smoothie	Garlic Mashed Potatoes & Turnips	Spicy Cheesy Tofu Balls	Honey Peanut Butter
11	Blueberry and chia smoothie	Green Beans with Bacon	Radish Chips	Mediterranean Marinated Olives
12	Green Kickstart Smoothie	Coconut Brussels Sprouts	Sautéed Pears	Nut Butter & Dates Granola

13	Warm Maple and Cinnamon Quinoa	Cod Stew with Rice & Sweet Potatoes	Pecan & Blueberry Crumble	Oven-baked Caramelize Plantains
14	Warm Quinoa Breakfast Bowl	Chicken & Rice	Rice Pudding	Powerful Peas & Lentils Dip
15	Banana Bread Rice Pudding	Rice Bowl with Edamame	Mango Sticky Rice	Protein "Raffaello" Candies
16	Apple and cinnamon oatmeal	Chickpea Avocado Sandwich	Noodles Alfredo with Herby Tofu	Protein-Rich Pumpkin Bowl
17	Mango Key Lime Pie Smoothie	Roasted Tomato Sandwich	Lemon Couscous with Tempeh Kabobs	Savory Red Potato-Garlic Balls
18	Spiced orange breakfast couscous	Pulled "Pork" Sandwiches	Portobello Burger with Veggie Fries	Spicy Smooth Red Lentil Dip

19	Breakfast parfaits	Cauliflower Latke	Thai Seitan Vegetable Curry	Steamed Broccoli with Sesame
20	Sweet potato and kale hash	Roasted Brussels Sprouts	Tofu Cabbage Stir-Fry	Vegan Eggplant Patties
21	Delicious Oat Meal	Brussels Sprouts & Cranberries Salad	Curried Tofu with Buttery Cabbage	Vegan Breakfast Sandwich
22	Breakfast Cherry Delight	Potato Latke	Smoked Tempeh with Broccoli Fritters	Chickpea And Mushroom Burger
23	Crazy Maple and Pear Breakfast	Broccoli Rabe	Cheesy Potato Casserole	Beans with Sesame Hummus
24	Hearty French Toast Bowls	Whipped Potatoes	Curry Mushroom Pie	Candied Honey-Coconut Peanuts
25	Chocolate PB Smoothie	Quinoa Avocado Salad	Spicy Cheesy Tofu Balls	Choco Walnuts Fat Bombs

26	Orange french toast	Roasted Sweet Potatoes	Radish Chips	Crispy Honey Pecans (Slow Cooker)
27	Oatmeal Raisin Breakfast Cookie	Cauliflower Salad	Sautéed Pears	Crunchy Fried Pickles
28	Berry Beetsicle Smoothie	Garlic Mashed Potatoes & Turnips	Pecan & Blueberry Crumble	Granola bars with Maple Syrup

Meal Plan 2

Day	Breakfast	Lunch	Dinner	Smoothie
1	Mexican-Spiced Tofu Scramble	Teriyaki Tofu Stir-fry	Mushroom Steak	Chocolate Smoothie
2	Whole Grain Protein Bowl	Red Lentil and Quinoa Fritters	Spicy Grilled Tofu Steak	Chocolate Mint Smoothie
3	Healthy Breakfast Bowl	Green Pea Fritters	Piquillo Salsa Verde Steak	Cinnamon Roll Smoothie
4	Healthy Breakfast Bowl	Breaded Tofu Steaks	Butternut Squash Steak	Coconut Smoothie
5	Root Vegetable Hash With Avocado Crème	Chickpea and Edamame Salad	Cauliflower Steak Kicking Corn	Maca Almond Smoothie
6	Chocolate Strawberry Almond Protein Smoothie	Thai Tofu and Quinoa Bowls	Pistachio Watermelon Steak	Blueberry Smoothie
7	Banana Bread Breakfast Muffins	Black Bean and Bulgur Chili	BBQ Ribs	Nutty Protein Shake

8	Stracciatella Muffins	Cauliflower Steaks	Spicy Veggie Steaks With veggies	Cinnamon Pear Smoothie
9	Cardamom Persimmon Scones With Maple-Persimmon Cream	Avocado and Hummus Sandwich	Mushroom Steak	Vanilla Milkshake
10	Activated Buckwheat & Coconut Porridge With Blueberry Sauce	Chickpea Spinach Salad	Spicy Grilled Tofu Steak	Raspberry Protein Shake
11	Sweet Molasses Brown Bread	Teriyaki Tofu Stir-fry	Piquillo Salsa Verde Steak	Raspberry Almond Smoothie
12	Mexican-Spiced Tofu Scramble	Red Lentil and Quinoa Fritters	Butternut Squash Steak	Chocolate Smoothie
13	Whole Grain Protein Bowl	Green Pea Fritters	Cauliflower Steak Kicking Corn	Chocolate Mint Smoothie
14	Healthy Breakfast Bowl	Breaded Tofu Steaks	Pistachio Watermelon Steak	Cinnamon Roll Smoothie

15	Healthy Breakfast Bowl	Chickpea and Edamame Salad	BBQ Ribs	Coconut Smoothie
16	Root Vegetable Hash With Avocado Crème	Thai Tofu and Quinoa Bowls	Spicy Veggie Steaks With veggies	Maca Almond Smoothie
17	Chocolate Strawberry Almond Protein Smoothie	Black Bean and Bulgur Chili	Mushroom Steak	Blueberry Smoothie
18	Banana Bread Breakfast Muffins	Cauliflower Steaks	Spicy Grilled Tofu Steak	Nutty Protein Shake
19	Stracciatella Muffins	Avocado and Hummus Sandwich	Piquillo Salsa Verde Steak	Cinnamon Pear Smoothie
20	Cardamom Persimmon Scones With Maple-Persimmon Cream	Chickpea Spinach Salad	Butternut Squash Steak	Vanilla Milkshake

21	Activated Buckwheat & Coconut Porridge With Blueberry Sauce	Teriyaki Tofu Stir-fry	Cauliflower Steak Kicking Corn	Raspberry Protein Shake
22	Sweet Molasses Brown Bread	Red Lentil and Quinoa Fritters	Pistachio Watermelon Steak	Raspberry Almond Smoothie
23	Mexican-Spiced Tofu Scramble	Green Pea Fritters	BBQ Ribs	Chocolate Smoothie
24	Whole Grain Protein Bowl	Breaded Tofu Steaks	Spicy Veggie Steaks With veggies	Chocolate Mint Smoothie
25	Healthy Breakfast Bowl	Chickpea and Edamame Salad	Mushroom Steak	Cinnamon Roll Smoothie
26	Healthy Breakfast Bowl	Thai Tofu and Quinoa Bowls	Spicy Grilled Tofu Steak	Coconut Smoothie
27	Root Vegetable Hash With Avocado Crème	Black Bean and Bulgur Chili	Piquillo Salsa Verde Steak	Maca Almond Smoothie

28	Chocolate Strawberry Almond Protein Smoothie	Cauliflower Steaks	Butternut Squash Steak	Blueberry Smoothie

Meal Plan 3

Day	Breakfast	Lunch	Dinner	Snacks
1	Breakfast Blueberry Muffins	Quinoa Buddha Bowl	Broccoli & black beans stir fry	Spiced Chickpeas
2	Oatmeal with Pears	Lettuce Hummus Wrap	Stuffed peppers	Lemon & Ginger Kale Chips
3	Yogurt with Cucumber	Simple Curried Vegetable Rice	Sweet 'n spicy tofu	Chocolate Energy Snack Bar
4	Breakfast Casserole	Spicy Southwestern Hummus Wraps	Eggplant & mushrooms in peanut sauce	Hazelnut & Maple Chia Crunch
5	Berries with Mascarpone on Toasted Bread	Buffalo Cauliflower Wings	Green beans stir fry	Roasted Cauliflower
6	Fruit Cup	Veggie Fritters	Collard greens 'n tofu	Apple Cinnamon Crisps
7	Oatmeal with Black Beans & Cheddar	Pizza Bites	Cassoulet	Pumpkin Spice Granola Bites

8	Breakfast Smoothie	Avocado, Spinach and Kale Soup	Double-garlic bean and vegetable soup	Salted Carrot Fries
9	Yogurt with Beets & Raspberries	Curry spinach soup	Mean bean minestrone	Zesty Orange Muffins
10	Curry Oatmeal	Arugula and Artichokes Bowls	Grilled Halloumi Broccoli Salad	Chocolate Tahini Balls
11	Fig & Cheese Oatmeal	Minty arugula soup	Black Bean Lentil Salad With Lime Dressing	Spiced Chickpeas
12	Pumpkin Oats	Spinach and Broccoli Soup	Arugula Lentil Salad	Lemon & Ginger Kale Chips
13	Sweet Potato Toasts	Coconut zucchini cream	Red Cabbage Salad With Curried Seitan	Chocolate Energy Snack Bar
14	Tofu Scramble Tacos	Zucchini and Cauliflower Soup	Chickpea, Red Kidney Bean And Feta Salad	Hazelnut & Maple Chia Crunch

15	Almond Chia Pudding	Chard soup	The Amazing Chickpea Spinach Salad	Roasted Cauliflower
16	Breakfast Parfait Popsicles	Avocado, Pine Nuts and Chard Salad	Curried Carrot Slaw With Tempeh	Apple Cinnamon Crisps
17	Strawberry Smoothie Bowl	Grapes, Avocado and Spinach Salad	Black & White Bean Quinoa Salad	Pumpkin Spice Granola Bites
18	Peanut Butter Granola	Greens and Olives Pan	Greek Salad With Seitan Gyros Strips	Salted Carrot Fries
19	Apple Chia Pudding	Mushrooms and Chard Soup	Chickpea And Edamame Salad	Zesty Orange Muffins
20	Pumpkin Spice Bites	Tomato, Green Beans and Chard Soup	Broccoli & black beans stir fry	Chocolate Tahini Balls
21	Lemon Spelt Scones	Hot roasted peppers cream	Stuffed peppers	Spiced Chickpeas
22	Veggie Breakfast Scramble	Eggplant and Peppers Soup	Sweet 'n spicy tofu	Lemon & Ginger Kale Chips

23	Breakfast Blueberry Muffins	Eggplant and Olives Stew	Eggplant & mushrooms in peanut sauce	Chocolate Energy Snack Bar
24	Oatmeal with Pears	Cauliflower and Artichokes Soup	Green beans stir fry	Hazelnut & Maple Chia Crunch
25	Yogurt with Cucumber	Quinoa Buddha Bowl	Collard greens 'n tofu	Roasted Cauliflower
26	Breakfast Casserole	Lettuce Hummus Wrap	Cassoulet	Apple Cinnamon Crisps
27	Berries with Mascarpone on Toasted Bread	Simple Curried Vegetable Rice	Double-garlic bean and vegetable soup	Pumpkin Spice Granola Bites
28	Fruit Cup	Spicy Southwestern Hummus Wraps	Mean bean minestrone	Salted Carrot Fries

Meal plan 4

Day	Breakfast	Entrées	Soup , Salad, & Sides	Smoothie
1	Tasty Oatmeal Muffins	Black Bean Dip	Spinach Soup with Dill and Basil	Fruity Smoothie
2	Omelet with Chickpea Flour	Cannellini Bean Cashew Dip	Coconut Watercress Soup	Energizing Ginger Detox Tonic
3	White Sandwich Bread	Cauliflower Popcorn	Coconut Watercress Soup	Warm Spiced Lemon Drink
4	A Toast to Remember	Cinnamon Apple Chips with Dip	Coconut Watercress Soup	Soothing Ginger Tea Drink
5	Tasty Panini	Crunchy Asparagus Spears	Cauliflower Spinach Soup	Nice Spiced Cherry Cider

6	Tasty Oatmeal and Carrot Cake	Cucumber Bites with Chive and Sunflower Seeds	Avocado Mint Soup	Fragrant Spiced Coffee
7	Onion & Mushroom Tart with a Nice Brown Rice Crust	Garlicky Kale Chips	Creamy Squash Soup	Tangy Spiced Cranberry Drink
8	Perfect Breakfast Shake	Hummus-stuffed Baby Potatoes	Cucumber Edamame Salad	Warm Pomegranate Punch
9	Beet Gazpacho	Homemade Trail Mix	Best Broccoli Salad	Rich Truffle Hot Chocolate
10	Vegetable Rice	Nut Butter Maple Dip	Rainbow Orzo Salad	Ultimate Mulled Wine
11	Courgette Risotto	Oven Baked Sesame Fries	Broccoli Pasta Salad	Pleasant Lemonade
12	Country Breakfast Cereal	Pumpkin Orange Spice Hummus	Eggplant & Roasted Tomato Farro Salad	Pineapple, Banana & Spinach Smoothie

13	Oatmeal Fruit Shake	Quick English Muffin Mexican Pizzas	Garden Patch Sandwiches on Multigrain Bread	Kale & Avocado Smoothie
14	Amaranth Banana Breakfast Porridge	Quinoa Trail Mix Cups	Garden Salad Wraps	Coconut & Strawberry Smoothie
15	Green Ginger Smoothie	Black Bean Dip	Marinated Mushroom Wraps	Pumpkin Chia Smoothie
16	Orange Dream Creamsicle	Cannellini Bean Cashew Dip	Tamari Toasted Almonds	Cantaloupe Smoothie Bowl
17	Strawberry Limeade	Cauliflower Popcorn	Nourishing Whole-Grain Porridge	Berry & Cauliflower Smoothie
18	Peanut Butter and Jelly Smoothie	Cinnamon Apple Chips with Dip	Pungent Mushroom Barley Risotto	Green Mango Smoothie

19	Banana Almond Granola	Crunchy Asparagus Spears	Spinach Soup with Dill and Basil	Chia Seed Smoothie
20	Tasty Oatmeal Muffins	Cucumber Bites with Chive and Sunflower Seeds	Coconut Watercress Soup	Mango Smoothie
21	Omelet with Chickpea Flour	Garlicky Kale Chips	Coconut Watercress Soup	Fruity Smoothie

Lightning Source UK Ltd.
Milton Keynes UK
UKHW021017030521
383041UK00001B/25